Skin Care

SECRETS REVEALED

WHAT WORKS & DOESN'T WORK

DISCOVER THE TOP SKIN CARE TIPS THAT WILL LEAVE YOU WITH CLEAR, BLEMISH-FREE, YOUTHFUL, VIBRANT, & REJUVENATED SKIN EVERYDAY

SAKURA VIOTTO

SKIN CARE

Secrets Revealed

Abundant Press - Las Vegas, NV 89107 www.AbundantPress.com

Special discounts are available on quantity purchases by corporations, associations, and others. For details, contact the publisher. Orders by U.S. & International trade bookstores and wholesalers at: info@abundantpress.com. Printed in the United States of America- Library of Congress-in-Publication Data. Please note: If you find errors, like spelling or grammar, please send us an email.

Author: Sakura Viotto

ISBN: 978-1-948287-27-2

.

Any product, website, and company names mentioned in this report are the trademarks or copyright properties of their respective owners. The author/publisher/reseller are not associated or affiliated with them in any way. Nor does the referred product, website, and company names sponsor, endorse, or approve this product.

Disclaimer

The information within this book is intended as reference material only and not as medical or professional advice. Information contained herein is intended to give you the tools to make informed decisions about your wellness, lifestyle, and physical and mental health. It should not be used as a substitute for any treatment that has been prescribed or recommended by your doctor. The information within this book must not be construed as a medical, therapeutic, or psychological treatment, nor are any such claims made.

Every reasonable effort has been made to ensure that the material within this book is true, correct, complete, and appropriate at the time of writing. Nevertheless, the authors do not accept responsibility for any omission or error, or for any injury, damage, loss, or financial consequences arising from the use of this material. The authors, promoters, and publishers are not healthcare professionals, and expressly disclaim any responsibility for any adverse effects occurring as a result of the use of the suggestions or information herein. This material is offered as practical, current information available about disease and health management for your own education and enjoyment.

If you suspect you have a disease of any kind, it is imperative that you seek medical attention. It is also recommended that you consult with a qualified healthcare professional before beginning any diet or exercise program. By accepting this information, you agree to hold Sakura Viotto, his associates, partners, and affiliates free of liability and damage, and you proceed on your own free will. You and you alone are solely responsible for the results that you produce. Do not continue unless you fully agree to these terms and conditions.

This constitutes the entire license agreement. Any disputes or terms not discussed in this agreement are at the sole discretion of the publisher. Important Note: It's important that you seek the advice and approval from your health care provider prior to making any drastic changes to your diet or exercise.

Sakura®
Nutraceuticals
ADVANCED PRODUCTS BACKED BY: NATURE+SCIENCE

For more information please visit:

www.SakuraNutraceuticals.com

Table of Contents

Introduction

It seems that more and more people are turning to natural skincare, and for a good reason. When you decide to use a natural skincare product as opposed to one that's commercially prepared, you're putting good things back into your body and saying no to harmful chemicals.

If you're considering taking on a new, more natural approach to your skincare routine, then we really think you'll enjoy this list of tips. We make it easy to get back to nature without having to spend a lot of money, time, or effort.

And we believe that by incorporating these natural skincare habits into your daily routine, that you'll both, feel and look your very best. So, if you want firmer skin, the ability to ward off bacterial infections without prescription medication, and to naturally turn back the clock on your eyes, then keep reading!

Important Note: It's important that you seek the advice and approval from your health care provider prior to making any drastic changes to your diet or exercise.

An Insider's Guide to Natural Skin Care

Natural skin care products may be the answer if you are concerned about the chemicals in most commercial cosmetic products. Some of these chemicals may be toxic enough to actually accelerate the aging process, which is the opposite of what you are trying to accomplish with your skin care. Even in these days of increased regulation and consumer watchdog groups, there are a number of new products introduced each year that still contain damaging chemicals.

Almost nine hundred toxic chemicals have been found in commercial cosmetic products by the National Institute of Occupational Safety and Health. The Cancer Coalition has stated that cosmetic and personal care products pose a higher threat of cancer than even smoking cigarettes. Compounding the problem is the vast amount of incorrect information distributed by marketing departments to attract new customers.

Everything that you put on the surface of your skin is absorbed into the pores and gets into the bloodstream. The circulation of the blood distributes the toxins throughout the entire body, causing damage to internal organs as well as the skin.

Since all of these products enter your body, you should analyze the labels on your cosmetic products the same way you would with labels on food. Of course, choosing only natural skin care products eliminates the problem of toxins altogether.

Once the toxins get into your bloodstream, it forces your body to work much harder than usual in an effort to get rid of them. The liver is responsible for most of this clean up, but it can only handle so much before health problems will set in. The liver is a key part of the body's immune system and should be treated with care. Liver problems can cause major health issues such as auto-immune diseases, asthma, continual infections, and allergies.

Using natural ingredients can avoid these toxicity problems. The body recognizes natural skin care products as organic matter to be processed, not as a toxic threat that must be eliminated. Many of these products are made out of plant matter which contains the same basic vitamins and minerals as the ones already present in our bodies. Synthetic chemicals may be seen by the body as toxic and the immune system will react against them.

You can exfoliate with a gentle material such as crushed oatmeal, table sugar, or baking soda. Make exfoliating a regular part of your daily skin care routine and you will see much more life and bounce in your appearance.

Other natural substances that may be useful for skin care include honey, egg whites, olive oil, bananas, and avocado. Be creative and use of some of the common items you have in your kitchen to give you softer, smoother skin.

How do you know which natural skin care products are actually safe? Some products are labeled as "100% natural" when they still contain chemicals and toxins.

The only way to be completely sure is to look at the list of ingredients on the package. Dyes, fragrances, and synthetic preservatives can all be found in these "natural" skin care products.

Sakura®
Nutraceuticals
ADVANCED PRODUCTS BACKED BY: NATURE+SCIENCE

www.SakuraNutraceuticals.com

Tip #1:
Rejuvenate Your Eyes

Our eyes love to show our current physical and mental state. This means that when you're exhausted, it's one of the first things that people around you will notice. Thanks to the power of caffeine though, you don't have to look too far for a natural way to de-puff your peepers!

So why do so many people turn to caffeine to brighten their eyes? There are several reasons, actually. First of all, caffeine brightens our skin and helps to remove those pesky dark circles. You know, the ones that like to hang out under our eyes.

In addition to decreasing the appearance of those dark circles, caffeine also helps our skin reduce inflammation when it's puffed up. Caffeine actually constricts the blood vessels right underneath our skin, and by doing so we get our regular skin tone back.

There are plenty of eye treatments on the market that promise to do all of this, but buyer beware. Steer clear of those with too many chemicals, and look for ones that are primarily made up of caffeine and B vitamins. Better yet, try this easy at-home remedy.

All you need to do is steep two, caffeinated tea bags in very hot water for about a minute or so. Then place both of them on a plate and put in your refrigerator to chill.

Once they're nice and cold, put one on each of your closed eyelids for up to 15 minutes. Voila! Goodbye tired eyes and hello, sunshine! To really see the difference, consider taking a before and after shot of your eyes.

Tip #2: Coconut Oil for Your Skin

Not only is coconut oil good for your physical health, but it also has many benefits when applied directly to your skin.

Coconut oil is high in good kinds of fat, which is why cooking with it is so beneficial. But those same fats also contain antimicrobial properties, which means they're great for your skin as well.

There are many different types of skin infections that you can develop; Athlete's foot and folliculitis are just a couple. By incorporating coconut oil into your natural skincare routine, your chances of developing a skin infection drastically diminishes.

More than half of the fatty acids in coconut oil are lauric acid, which is extremely antimicrobial and helps ward off nasty bacteria. In fact, studies have shown it to be one of the best fatty acids to prevent bacterial infections.

You can easily incorporate coconut oil into your natural skincare by using it as a body moisturizer, hair mask, and even as a facial moisturizer.

It's important to keep your skin type in mind before trying coconut oil, though, as it can clog your pores. Start by using it on a small patch of your skin and see how you react. If you're unsure of your skin type, then consult with a physician who can make that determination with you.

Make sure to always opt for the all-natural variety to avoid adding any extra unneeded chemicals to your skin.

Tip #3: Natural Facelifts

As we get older, our skin slowly loses its elasticity. This leads to a sagging face that can reflect our true age, sometimes even making us look older than we really are. But you don't have to spend a penny to fix this common skincare concern.

Yoga is an ancient form of stretching that thousands of people practice on a daily basis. In addition to keeping our joints intact and strong, there are certain moves that will give you an instant facelift.

Before having your picture taken or going to a big event, take a few minutes and practice one or more of the following yoga poses:

Downward-Facing Dog: Start in plank position like you're getting ready to do a pushup. Slowly bring your rear and abdomen upward, making an upside down v with your body. Hold this pose for several seconds and then move back into plank position.

Deep Forward Fold: Standing straight, keep your feet firmly planted as you lean forward, letting your hands fall straight in front of you. Hold for one to five minutes, and then slowly come back up. To stretch your shoulders, fold your arms, grabbing your elbows and gently sway your torso from side to side.

Bridge Pose: Laying on your back with your feet stretched out in front of you and your hands behind your head, slowly lift and arch your back until the top of your head is touching the ground. Hold for one to five minutes, and then slowly lower yourself back down.

As with any physical activity, please check with your healthcare provider ahead of time.

All of these movements increase blood circulation to your face, along with giving it a temporary facelift.

Yet another reason to start practicing yoga!

Tip #4:
Calming Green Algae

If you think back to your middle school days, specifically when you were learning about chlorophyll, you probably remember playing with algae. Well, there's a reason to start playing with it again, as an adult: natural skincare!

Chlorella vulgaris, which is the scientific word for algae, is chockfull of beta carotene and lutein, which are minerals that your body needs. Beta carotene is an anti-aging miracle nutrient, thanks to the high levels of antioxidants. No wonder your parents made you eat so many carrots as a kid!

But what is lutein, and why is it good for you?

More than ever, we are feeling our deep connection to one another. Cell phones, tablets, computers, and technological advancements leave your loved ones at the touch of a button. Chances are, you spend a good amount of your day staring at some type of screen.

That can show in your eyes.

Lutein works as a barrier from blue light exposure for your eyes, which is exactly the type of light that hits you when you stare at screens. In addition to being used as a natural barrier, it also does double duty for your skin.

This amazing antioxidant actually increases both skin hydration and elasticity!

The benefits of algae in terms of skincare:

1. Detoxifying
2. Moisturizing
3. Reduces fine lines and wrinkles

And the best part is, algae isn't specific to just one type of skin. Which means that it doesn't matter if yours is oily or dry, you can still reap the benefits.

While there are plenty of natural skincare products that contain algae, consider buying some powdered algae and making your own face mask at home.

Just mix 1/4 cup of the powder with, either 2 tablespoons of olive oil (for dry skin), or 2 tablespoons of clay (for oily skin. Add your favorite essential oil, some water, and apply to your clean face. Relax for 20 minutes and then rinse off.

Make this a regular part of your skincare routine to see the long-term benefits of algae!

Tip #5: Stay Hydrated

We hear it all the time: drinking water is so important, and for good reason. Our body is made up of more than 50% water, which we lose throughout the day when we perspire. But it's not just our internal body that takes a hit when we become dehydrated.

It shows in our face, too.

Unlike sugar-laden soda and drinks filled with chemicals, pure water helps to flush out toxins within our body. Those toxins can wreak havoc to our skin, causing uneven skin tones and loss of elasticity.

Furthermore, our blood needs somewhere to look when it gets low in water and becomes dehydrated. That's when it leeches onto skin cells and sucks up all of that water, which can often result in dark eye circles and deep eye sockets.

If you've ever eaten something that's high in sodium, such as pretzels, then you know how it feels to retain water. Because that's what sodium does. And when we retain water, it can often show in our skin.

Drinking plenty of water not only helps get rid of that bloat, but it also helps get rid of the puffiness that accompanies water retention.

And if you've ever experienced acne as an adult, then you'll want to consider drinking even more water. Some of the toxins that contribute to adult acne can easily be flushed away with higher water intake.

As you can see, you don't need to invest in expensive skincare or necessarily give up your favorite salty snack. Just try sneaking in a little more water, then watch and feel your skin get back to its glory days!

Tip #6: Exercise, Meditation and Sleep

While taking care of your body has some obvious benefits for your physical health, you might be surprised to know just how much it affects your skin too. And that includes keeping stress at bay.

When you go to bed after a long day, your main goal is to recharge your internal clock. But what you might not know, is that as that's happening, your skin is naturally rejuvenating itself. So not only do you need a good night's sleep to physically function, but your skin needs it too!

To ensure that you rest long enough every night, make sure to maintain a peaceful and relaxing bedroom atmosphere. Turn off all mobile devices and invest in a good mattress. Try reading before you go to bed instead of watching television.

In addition to getting a good night's sleep, it's imperative to have a solid and healthy exercise routine, and not just for your physical health. By regularly exercising, you're getting rid of stress and releasing endorphins. Getting rid of stress means getting rid of toxins, which can cause your skin to look and feel lackluster.

Before starting an exercise routine, be sure to meet with your physician.

Another great stress reliever is meditation. When we relax and calm our minds, focusing only on our breathing, we tend to look at everything around us in a brand new light. Having a more positive outlook means less stress on our bodies, which equates to an overall healthy glow.

If you make all three of these changes as part of your new, natural skincare routine, you'll be surprised at how much better you look and feel in just a short amount of time. When you feel good on the inside, it shows on the outside!

Tip #7:
Tea Tree Oil

You've probably heard about the many benefits of tea tree oil, which is derived from Melaleuca Alternifolia, also known as, Tea Trees. They are full of medicinal properties. It's no wonder that so many people keep a bottle on hand and the essential oil movement is on the rise!

Tea Tree oil is great for soothing dry skin, and its natural antiseptic qualities help combat oily skin as well. So, if you have either dry or oily skin, look for a natural lotion that contains real tea tree oil. It's important that it be diluted, since Tea Tree oil is so potent.

If you have itchy skin, consider applying some directly to the affected area. You'll want to dilute with a carrier oil, though. It's recommended that you use 12 drops of another oil to every two or three drops of Tea Tree. And being very antibacterial means it's perfect for healing wounds stemming from bacterial infections.

Tea Tree oil is also great for treating boils, which often occur from skin rubbing together and getting overheated. Treat the infected area by diluting some Tea Tree oil with water, dabbing it on a cotton swab and applying it to the boil two or three times per day. It will slowly cause the boil to come to a head and begin to heal.

Be sure to keep the surrounding area of your skin clean by applying a washcloth, since you don't want to spread the infection onto. What will come out will be a mixture of blood and puss, and it's best to keep that contained. Once properly drained, apply a bandage and change it daily until fully healed.

You can find Tea Tree oil in whole foods stores and medicinal shops, along with many online retailers.

Tip #8: Limes

When you think of limes, you probably think of tropical drinks or lemon-lime soda. But this popular citrus fruit is actually very beneficial for your skin.

If you have any dark spots on your skin that you'd like to brighten, then invest in some limes and cotton balls. Simply take a bit of lime juice, dip a cotton ball in it, and apply it to the affected area for about a half an hour.

This same technique can help fade scars and pimple markings, thanks to its natural bleaching agent. And if you suffer from loose skin, then good news: it helps with that, too!

In addition to all the above, lime juice is also full of antibiotic properties that help inhibit the growth of acne-causing bacteria.

You don't have to lime juice directly to the skin to reap its benefits, though.

Your skin can still get a glow from it by drinking the following concoction: the juice of one lime, a tablespoon of honey, and eight ounces of lukewarm water mixed together, every morning. The natural bleaching properties will help give your skin an overall glow.

Consider using lime peel as a scrub, too. There are plenty of easy, at-home recipes that call for just a few easy to find ingredients, plus lime peel, which will save you from applying chemicals found in commercially made face scrubs. Natural skincare, for the win!

Tip #9: Shea Butter

Shea butter is popping up everywhere nowadays. The next time you're at the store, take a look at the skincare aisle and notice how many lotions contain this natural moisturizer.

It's popular for many reasons, one of them being that it encourages natural collagen production.

Collagen is what our skin needs to feel full and lustrous, filling out those fine lines and wrinkles. And it's perfect for all skin types, which means you can reap the benefits whether your skin is dry, combination, or oily!

Shea butter also melts at body temperature, which makes it perfect for absorbing in through our pores. Like some other items mentioned on here, it's also high in fatty acids that our skin needs.

An amazing compound found in shea butter is phenolic, which protects skin from free radicals. Loosely translated, that means that it's anti-aging, which is a big plus when it comes to natural skincare. When used regularly, it can also help to prevent stretch marks!

There are plenty of natural shea butter lotions that you can buy, but you can also purchase pure shea butter and apply it directly to your skin.

Just remember to try and avoid as many harsh chemicals as possible when buying anything that you're going to put on-or in-your body. It deserves the best!

Tip #10: Facial Steaming

You've probably seen pictures and videos of women getting steamy facials. It's a popular procedure at beauty salons for many reasons. But don't worry, you don't have to loosen the purse strings too much to get one yourself.

Steaming your face opens your pores, which means it loosens all of that built-up gunk and dirt. It also gets rid of acne-causing bacteria as well. It opens your pores, which is great if you suffer from millia: small, white bumps on your face that are full of oil.

Steaming your face also warms up the surface for any facial treatments you'll be getting, which is why estheticians like to do it before applying face masks. And it also enhances circulation, which is perfect for maintaining a youthful glow.

To do an at-home steaming session, simply boil some water, place in a heatproof bowl, drape a towel over your neck, and steam for 10-15 minutes before patting dry.

If you feel like splurging, you can also buy an at-home facial steamer and use that instead. Whichever you prefer, just so long as you steam your face and open those pores!

Conclusion

As you can now see, it doesn't take a whole lot to incorporate natural skincare into your daily routine. By simply consuming more water, getting plenty of rest, and trying these natural tips, you'll soon be on your way to looking and feeling great.

When searching for additional supplements for your natural skincare routine, whether oral or topical, remember to limit the number of chemicals that you put into your body. The more natural you can be, the better it'll be for you in the long run.

As with any new program, be sure to consult with your physician before making any major new changes, especially when it comes to physical activity.

We wish you the very best on your new journey toward a more natural skincare routine!

Benefits of Natural Beauty Secrets

Women everywhere around the world are literally dying to know natural beauty secrets. As women go under the knife for one plastic surgery after another, they risk their lives and their bodies in an attempt to appear naturally beautiful. Little thought is given to how a botched surgery can affect them or their loved ones down the road. All they can think of is this unrealistic image of what's considered beautiful that they have in the heads thanks to the media and advertising.

The truth is, natural beauty secrets are not really all that secret. Everywhere a woman looks, she can find all natural ways to become someone that is truly beautiful instead of trying to imitate a digitally airbrushed and otherwise changed photograph from an ad in a magazine. A couple of the biggest secrets entail nothing more than loving yourself for precisely who you are, perceived imperfections and all.

There are so many benefits of natural beauty secrets. If you make the decision to love yourself for exactly who you are and make an effort to do so daily, your self-confidence will soar.

If you are happy with who you are, you will be a happier person.

If you're a happier person, your interactions with others will be more pleasant. If you treat others more kindly, they will also be happier. The world could literally be a better place if women decided to love themselves; instead of aspiring to be something no normal woman could ever be.

Everyone wants a better quality of life. For some women, they feel that if they just looked like that model or such-and-such celebrity, they would have everything they could possibly want and more. They feel that sort of beauty will open doors for them. In reality, while beauty might open a few doors, those doors will quickly be shut if you're ugly on the inside. A woman who is dedicated to getting what she wants and feels she deserves will go much farther in this world than one who relies on her good looks alone.

Another benefit of the natural beauty secret of being happy with who you are is, at the end of the day, when all is said and done, you only have yourself. If you don't like yourself as a person, you can't expect anyone else to like you, either.

While some may immediately be drawn to you because of your perceived beauty, they will quickly leave once they realize how poisonous your personality is. You'll wind up alone, with only a mirror for company.

Stop letting others dictate what you should wear, how you should look, or how you should act! Don't let people who don't even know you tell you what to do with your life and body! The media and advertising executives don't know who you are.

They don't even know you exist. Make the choice to do what's best for you. That is the real natural beauty secret.

Discover the Truth About All-Natural Beauty

All-natural beauty is something many women want but few know they have. Instead, they get expensive surgeries done, literally risking their lives in the pursuit of a beauty standard that is not only unrealistic but is completely unreal. They use beauty products that damage their skin and hair and ultimately wind up in landfills when they don't have the promised effects. Women are hurting themselves and the environment all in an effort to be beautiful.

Fortunately, there are many different ways women can achieve the all-natural beauty that they so desperately want and deserve. Some of these ways are exceptionally easy to incorporate into a woman's everyday life. Some of them may be a little bit trickier for some to get used to doing everyday but once fitted into a woman's daily habits, they will be easy to maintain for a lifetime.

The first step to all natural beauty is to stop idolizing the models you see in magazines or on billboards. Stop looking to female celebrities and comparing yourself to them.

Nearly all advertisements in magazines, billboards, even head shots used in portfolios, have been touched up in one way or another digitally to get rid of wrinkles, acne, or other unsightly blemishes.

No woman can ever live up to how a model looks in a photo because the photo simply isn't real.

Next, women everywhere need to realize how beautiful they already are. Everyone has flaws or imperfections that they don't like about themselves; even models and celebrities. You need to quit focusing on where you think you don't measure up and instead focus on things you like about yourself. For some women, finding things they appreciate about themselves can be a difficult task. Recruit friends and loved ones to tell you what they like about you. You don't have to restrict yourself to looks, either.

Which leads to the next truth about all-natural beauty: it comes from within. It may sound very cliche but the phrase has existed for a long time for a reason. Beautiful personalities, feeling confident in yourself without being cocky, helping others, and honestly caring for those around you will make you a truly beautiful person. People with picture perfect bodies but who have ugly hearts and souls may lead a charmed life on the outside but on the inside; things aren't as lovely.

Because they are so mean and hurtful to those around them, they drive people away from them, and wind up alone in the end.

Surround yourself with people that are truly beautiful from the inside and you will not only be happier but you'll stop turning to a Hollywood standard that even models and celebrities can't live up to. Don't be tempted to turn into a plastic person through plastic surgery or other extreme measures in order to be a fantasy version of someone who doesn't know you exist. The truth about all-natural beauty is in understanding the beauty within.

How to Choose the Right Skin Care Products

The right set of skin care products can show the world that you care about your appearance and what you use on your skin. After all, your face is the first thing people see when they meet you, so you want to look your best. Here are some things to look for when trying to protect your skin.

Simply washing your face with soap alone is not sufficient daily skin care. Soap may clean up some of the oil and dirt on your face and may even open up some pores, but it does nothing to moisturize or condition your skin. In addition to your normal daily routine of washing with soap, add in some quality skin care products to protect and soften your skin.

There are a number of facial care products on the market to choose from. Always use a facial cleanser instead of regular bar soap because body soap can dry out the face and will not give you any of the moisturizing properties of a good cleanser. Specially designed cleansers can be used for treating oily or dry skin, soothing sensitive skin, removing acne, or cleaning off cosmetics. Facial cleansers are available in different varieties, such as liquid, foam, cream, or gel.

You can also find a selection of face lotions in any line of skin care products. These are usually much lighter than the heavy body lotions because they must moisturize while also controlling oily skin.

Many of these lotions also give you other benefits like tanning, wrinkle prevention, or sunblock. These are all important if you want to protect your youthful appearance and stave off wrinkles.

Always take care of your face each day, starting off by cleansing to remove built up dirt and oil. This will make sure your pores stay open and clear, preventing acne. The proper skin care products can help you get rid of all that accumulated dirt, oil, and pollutants from the air that may have built up on your face. Leaving this untreated may lead to more serious skin problems or even infection if the buildup is too great.

Specialized skin care products are also available to deal with conditions like eczema, blackheads, and whiteheads. There are wipes, pads, gels, creams, foams, and more that are all individually designed to handle a certain skin condition. To clean out the pores overnight, you can get a facial mask that hardens on the skin and peels off with all of the impurities. Check the instructions that come with the product as some require the mask to be rinsed off and others simply can be peeled off.

For more luxurious skin care treatment, you can go to a spa for a full-service facial. In addition to facial services, most spas offer body massages and saunas so you can also unwind and reduce stress. While these high-end services may be expensive, you can usually get a basic facial for a reasonable price at most spas. Also, a quality spa should have the latest in skin care products for you to purchase for your own home use.

Natural Beauty Tips to Help You Look Your Best

Let our natural beauty tips help you look beautiful without all those toxic chemicals found in today's cosmetics. It is possible to achieve a healthy, vibrant appearance using only natural ingredients. You'll look better and feel better because you do not have all those heavy cosmetic products on your skin.

Natural beauty refers to a vital and healthy look for your body, hair, and skin. Living an overall healthier lifestyle is the first step to refreshing your appearance. Take care of your body from the inside out before attempting to fix skin problems with surface treatments like moisturizer or makeup. Many times, a simple lifestyle change is all it takes to completely revitalize your look.

Make sure you are eating right and are getting enough vitamins and minerals each day. Add a multivitamin to your morning routine to ensure that you are receiving all the nutrients your body needs. Eat plenty of fruits and vegetables and try to avoid excess fats, sugars, and processed foods. Healthy food for your body will show through in your appearance as your skin clears and becomes more moist and supple.

Exercise is probably the most powerful of any of the natural beauty tips. Regular physical activity improves blood flow to the skin, giving it a fuller, more colorful look naturally. Of course, exercise will also help you stay trim and looking good all-around. On top of the benefits to your appearance, working out on a regular basis will keep your internal organs and heart healthy, along with preventing some cancers and extending your life.

The next in our list of natural beauty tips is to always keep yourself hydrated. As skin dries out, it becomes inflexible and more susceptible to wrinkles. Instead of applying heavy moisturizing cream externally, try drinking more water to provide moisture from the inside. This is a far healthier and natural solution to the common problem of dry skin.

Even if you still want to wear some cosmetics, there are natural beauty tips that can help you. Start off with either a sheer foundation or a slightly tinted moisturizing cream. Use a damp sponge to apply the cream so you get coverage all over your face without too much cosmetic buildup. This shows off your healthy-looking skin, but will also cover up any blemishes or marks without being too heavy or obvious.

To avoid leathery, dry skin, stay out of the sun whenever possible. The UV rays from the sun will dry out your skin and cause it to wrinkle prematurely. If you must go out in direct sunlight, be sure to wear sunscreen that is rated SPF 15 or higher. Hats, sunglasses, and umbrellas can also help protect you when you are out in the sun.

As you can see it does not require chemical-filled cosmetics and makeup to look great. There are many ways to enhance your appearance without resorting to artificial products. Following these natural beauty tips will get you on your way to a healthier, more radiant appearance.

Proven Techniques for Natural Health and Beauty Recipes

The green movement and global warming have people everywhere in search of natural health and beauty recipes. As more and more people discover these all-natural recipes, more and more people decide to make them at home instead of spending the money to buy similar products from the various beauty and health stores. Who can blame them? These sorts of products tend to be more expensive than their toxic counterparts. If you make them at home, you'll save money and the environment.

Part of the problem is, as most people embark down the path of making natural health and beauty recipes, they have little to no experience in making them. People can then become discouraged and give up trying to make them at home, finding it easier and cheaper to just go back to their old, planet destroying habits. Before you throw in the towel, there are several techniques that can help give a successful result on any of the recipes you try.

Actually, the first thing anyone should do when deciding to make any of the natural health and beauty recipes they find is to do some research. The internet is a great resource in learning about the ingredients used in the recipes and where to find them.

You can also find tips and tricks from people who have made the recipe before, allowing you to learn from their experience and mistakes before you attempt to make it yourself. Why learn the hard way and make your own mistakes when you can learn from someone else's?

Next, you'll want to purchase a good reference book on natural health and beauty recipes. It's not always possible to hop on the internet and look up the information you need when you're right in the middle of creating something. A good reference book is also great for researching any particular ailments that might spring up on you suddenly. Having one on essential oils is a must since essential oils are used quite frequently in these sorts of recipes.

Since quite a few natural health and beauty recipes are cooked much like regular, food recipes, you'll want to purchase separate cook wear that will be used when you make your beauty recipes. Some ingredients can do wonders for a complexion but cause serious problems if ingested. It can be hard to get a pot completely clean and free of any essential oil or plant residue once it's been used for a beauty recipe. You'll avoid the likelihood of cross-contamination all together if you simply use different cook wear for different things.

When you're ready to make one of the beauty recipes, gather all of your ingredients and the recipe together, much like when you cook normally. Make sure you keep your work area clean and wipe up any spills immediately. Have whatever containers ready that you plan on storing your creation in. Natural health and beauty recipes aren't hard to do. They can be a lot of fun!

The Benefits of Professional Skin Care

You can get a variety of professional skin care products just about anywhere these days. It used to be that you were limited to only the selection of products at your local spa, but now there are quality skin care products at the pharmacy or health store, along with a number of outlets online. You no longer have to pay expensive spa fees just to get the products you need.

Along with the expanded choice of retailers, there is a vast array of professional skin care products available. You can choose an entire product line to cover all of your personal care needs or just select single products as you need them.

There are also more organic and natural beauty products on the market now than ever before, so you do not have to use chemical-based skin care products. Some products have blended the natural with some synthetic substances, trying to avoid using the most toxic chemicals.

Many of these products can be purchased over the counter with no prescription, but some of the stronger items may require a prescription from a dermatologist. These products are usually a stronger concentration that is meant only for certain skin problems.

They must be restricted because they may cause damage to people who do not have that particular condition. Some of the more common prescription products are used to treat acne, discoloration, and premature aging.

Of course, if you do need a prescription product, you will have to make an appointment with a dermatologist. A qualified dermatologist is the best person to decide if you have a severe enough skin condition to warrant treatment with professional skin care products. If he does determine that you have a problem, the dermatologist can suggest certain products that will be best suited for that specific skin condition. The doctor can also advise you on the safe use of all cosmetic products, including warnings specific to pregnant women.

Any professional skin care product you buy should come with an instruction booklet and warnings. A good dermatologist will also verbally warn you of any side effect and should explain how to use the product correctly. Always follow the doctor's instructions or ask the pharmacist if you have any questions about how the product should be used or how much to use.

Although all professional skin care products come with their own instruction leaflets, your dermatologist should be able to verbally repeat product instructions and warnings.

A good doctor will always warn you if you should expect some side effects. He can also tell you exactly how to safely get the most out of your product. You should also check with your doctor to make sure there are no adverse reactions with any other medications or products you are currently using.

The expansion of the skin care industry has brought many high-end products to the consumer. You may now be able to find your skin care solution without having to see the dermatologist. Of course, be careful when purchasing your own products without a doctor's guidance as there may be side effects or interactions. Always do your research to make sure you are getting the right type of professional skin care products.

The Professionals Guide to Sensitive Skin Care

Sensitive skin care is a challenge for many people, especially those living in difficult climates. There are certain external conditions that should be avoided, as should the chemicals in most commercial cosmetic products. How do you know if you have sensitive skin? Here are a few factors to consider when deciding if you need specialized sensitive skin care products:

- Do you break out or have redness after being exposed to environmental stressors like shaving or weather?
- Do you have tingly or tight skin with no other explanation for it?
- Have you noticed any dryness, irritation, or redness on your skin?
- Does your skin react adversely to household cleaning products or cosmetics?
- After answering the rest of these questions, has your dermatologist ruled out any other skin conditions that could be causing the problem?

Sensitive skin can be even more challenging to deal with in adverse weather conditions.

If you live where the weather is extremely cold or hot, you may need to use sensitive skin care products to protect yourself.

Thin skin is generally more sensitive than thicker parts of the skin simply because there is less protection between the blood and the outside conditions. The capillaries are closer to the outside of the skin when it is thin, so the skin becomes sensitive to cold, heat, and wind. Sensitive skin also is more susceptible to sunburn, so wear a higher SPF sunscreen if you much go out in the sun.

Avoid harsh washing products like loofahs, brushes, or cleansing stones. You want something soft to take care of your sensitive skin, not an abrasive brush that will further irritate it. Do not use exfoliants because they may be too rough for your skin and cause inflammation when used.

Stay away from any strong chemicals in your skin care products. Fragrances and dyes in particular may irritate sensitive skin, so look for hypo-allergenic or organic products whenever possible. Use liquid cleansers as they are usually easier on the skin and will not cause the same allergic reactions. Hard-milled soaps also work well for sensitive skin care.

Antibacterial astringents are another key component of a good sensitive skin care program. They come in both cream and lotion form and are used to protect your skin from infectious bacteria. This balances your skin growth and keeps bacterial colonies from forming on the surface.

One strong antibacterial is salicylic acid, which can exfoliate and remove the outer layer of accumulated dead skin cells. It also clears out bacteria in hair follicle areas to ensure healthy hair growth.

Be careful when purchasing your sensitive skin care products to make sure that they really are safe for your skin. Many products are labeled as natural or hypo-allergenic when they still contain toxic chemicals.

Always check the ingredients listed on the label to see if there are any substances that may aggravate your skin. Similarly, perfume-free products may not always be completely devoid of fragrances so double-check all of your sensitive skin care products before use.

Where to Find the Latest Skin Care Information

There is so much skin care information out there today that it can be a bit perplexing to make sense of it all. This article will show you where to look to find the most accurate information and how to use that information to make a decision on your skin care products.

Look at the label on the product itself first. Most of the time, you can find all the information you need right there on the bottle. Cosmetic products are required to list all of the active ingredients and frequently will also list what each ingredient does. If you need more information, you can then research each of these ingredients individually to find out if there are any harmful effects.

To find out if there have been any allergic reactions or consumer problems with a certain product, check any of the skin care information websites on the Internet. Many times, you can find a message board or product review site where people are sharing their own individual experience with the product. Keep in mind that it is often the most dissatisfied customers who post on such sites, not customers who were happy with their purchase. Do not automatically write off a product that has had bad reviews, but you should at least do a little more research before buying.

You can also use the Internet to look up drug interactions or possible side effects. There are many medical websites available for general information. Of course, you should always check with a doctor if you have any preexisting medical conditions that may pose a serious danger. Internet skin care information can still be unreliable and you would not want to take a risk based on some anonymous person's opinion.

Your friends and family can also be a great source for skin care information. Simply ask around to find out if anyone has stumbled onto a great new skin care product. Pay particular attention to any of your friends who have undergone a major appearance overhaul as it is likely that they have tried out at least one of the skin care products on the market. If the product causes irritation or other side effects, your friend can also pass on her valuable experience and save you some hassle and pain.

If you need expert skin care information, contact a dermatologist. They often have stores of experience with their patients to draw from, so they can tell you if a certain product really works or if it is just marketing hype. They also should know about any dangerous side effects or drug interactions, so it is always a good idea to double-check with a dermatologist before starting any new skin care program.

Always research any new product before beginning to use it, especially if you have any other medical conditions. With all the resources available, there is no reason to take an unnecessary risk because you are uninformed. There is a lot of skin care information out there, it's just a matter of knowing where to look for it.

An Insider's Guide to Natural Skin Care

Natural skin care products may be the answer if you are concerned about the chemicals in most commercial cosmetic products. Some of these chemicals may be toxic enough to actually accelerate the aging process, which is the opposite of what you are trying to accomplish with your skin care. Even in these days of increased regulation and consumer watchdog groups, there are a number of new products introduced each year that still contain damaging chemicals.

Almost nine hundred toxic chemicals have been found in commercial cosmetic products by the National Institute of Occupational Safety and Health. The Cancer Coalition has stated that cosmetic and personal care products pose a higher threat of cancer than even smoking cigarettes. Compounding the problem is the vast amount of incorrect information distributed by marketing departments to attract new customers.

Everything that you put on the surface of your skin is absorbed into the pores and gets into the bloodstream.

The circulation of the blood distributes the toxins throughout the entire body, causing damage to internal organs as well as the skin.

Since all of these products enter your body, you should analyze the labels on your cosmetic products the same way you would with labels on food. Of course, choosing only natural skin care products eliminates the problem of toxins altogether.

Once the toxins get into your bloodstream, it forces your body to work much harder than usual in an effort to get rid of them. The liver is responsible for most of this clean up, but it can only handle so much before health problems will set in. The liver is a key part of the body's immune system and should be treated with care. Liver problems can cause major health issues such as auto-immune diseases, asthma, continual infections, and allergies.

Using natural ingredients can avoid these toxicity problems. The body recognizes natural skin care products as organic matter to be processed, not as a toxic threat that must be eliminated.

Many of these products are made out of plant matter which contains the same basic vitamins and minerals as the ones already present in our bodies. Synthetic chemicals may be seen by the body as toxic and the immune system will react against them.

You can exfoliate with a gentle material such as crushed oatmeal, table sugar, or baking soda. Make exfoliating a regular part of your daily skin care routine and you will see much more life and bounce in your appearance.

Other natural substances that may be useful for skin care include honey, egg whites, olive oil, bananas, and avocado. Be creative and use of some of the common items you have in your kitchen to give you softer, smoother skin.

How do you know which natural skin care products are actually safe? Some products are labeled as "100% natural" when they still contain chemicals and toxins.

The only way to be completely sure is to look at the list of ingredients on the package. Dyes, fragrances, and synthetic preservatives can all be found in these "natural" skin care products.

Case Study: Hydroderm vs. Other Skin Care

Wondering about the performance of Hydroderm vs. other skin care methods? In the past, there were few alternatives to hide the signs of aging. You were often limited to wearing scarves or neckties to cover up baggy neck lines and loose skin around the collar. Now there are a number of surgical procedures and cosmetic products on the market to take care of these unsightly problems. This article will explore how these new methods stack up against Hydroderm skin care products.

Chemical peels are one of the more common skin care methods being used today. A chemical peel actually burns off the top layer of skin with acid to remove the dead skin cells and let the healthy layer underneath shine through. This is a popular choice because it is non-invasive and does not require surgery. Chemical peels may not be as effective as a surgical procedure like a face life, but they are a good way to remove acne scars or sun damage.

Botox is one of the latest skin care methods to hit the marketplace. It uses small injections of collagen around the mouth, neck, or eye area to relax the muscles and reduce lines and wrinkling. It is also commonly used for people who have issues with involuntary muscle contraction, along with helping to smooth appearance.

Botox injections are commonly administered into the neck area, making them non-invasive and easy to recover from.

One of the oldest methods of taking years of one's appearance is the face lift. This is a much more involved, and often painful, surgical procedure in which the skin is actually cut and then tightened. Obviously, this is more costly than any of the other methods listed, including Hydroderm. A face lift may also require an extended recovery period to heal from the incisions that have been made.

Hydroderm is a new collagen infusion that is designed to moisturize the skin and tighten up wrinkles and lines. It is generally used in the neck area to pick up sagging skin. Hydroderm includes tri-dimensional proteins that fortify and revitalize dry, baggy skin. It is also currently the only way to infuse collagen into your system without painful injections at the doctor's office.

Hydroderm compares favorably vs. other skin care methods like the face lift, chemical peel, or Botox. In three weeks of the Hydroderm system, you can eliminate about half of the wrinkles on your face and neck. Even better, this does not require any surgery or injections and can be done in the privacy of your own home.

There are more options for skin care treatment than ever before. So far, Hydroderm holds its own vs. other skin care methods. It is far more economical and convenient than having a surgical procedure such as a face lift or an injection of Botox. It remains to be seen how Hydroderm will fare vs. other new skin care methods as they appear on the market, but right now it is still one of the best alternatives available.

Discover the Truth about All-Natural Health and Beauty Products

It seems that everywhere you turn nowadays, someone is selling new all natural health and beauty products. It seems that as more and more news coverage is aired or printed about global warming and the green movement, more and more business are trying to jump on the bandwagon in an effort to sell more products to consumers. It can be so hard to know what to think or who to believe when there's so much conflicting information going around.

As one might guess, the truth about all natural health and beauty products is that they all aren't created equal. Some products are better than others. Some products work and some don't. Some products are less harmful to the environment and some are flat out bad for the environment that everyone seems intent on saving. How is someone to know who to believe and who not to believe?

With money being tighter than ever, it's impossible to try out all of the available products to see for ourselves which actually do what they claim to. Fortunately, for some products, you won't have to. All you need to do is look through the ingredient list of your favorite products to get an idea for which ones are truly all natural and which ones aren't.

Perhaps one of the all-natural health and beauty products that can have the most impact, especially for women, is make-up. Mineral make-up is all the rage these days, it seems. But, as can be expected, not all mineral make-up is the same. While all boast being made from all natural minerals, they don't have to be made up entirely of just minerals. Many of the all-natural mineral brands include preservatives and other artificial ingredients to prolong the shelf life of the make-up. As we all know, preservatives and artificial ingredients can be harmful not just to ourselves but to the environment, as well.

Besides make-up, there are other all natural health and beauty products available for people to buy today. Shampoos, soaps, perfumes, even ointments for aching joints, can all carry the all-natural label. Once again, it's important to actually read the ingredients list to find out whether they are truly 100% natural. If there's a long, highly technical term in the ingredients list that you can't pronounce, chances are the product contains artificial stabilizers or preservatives. If you're truly wanting to go all natural, you'll definitely want to avoid those kinds of products.

Purchasing and using all natural health and beauty products is an excellent way to do something great for ourselves and for the environment. All natural products are safer for those with severe allergies as there is less of a chance someone might be allergic to them. Many of the beauty products come from renewable sources which lessens the strain on the environment. You can feel good about making yourself look good every day when you use all natural health and beauty products.

Discover Tips About Natural Beauty Products

With so many dangerous chemicals in mainstream cosmetics these days, more and more women are turning to the idea of natural beauty. Natural beauty is the practice of using only organic ingredients for skin and hair care. This avoids many of the health and allergy issues caused by commercial personal care products. Here are a few tips on how to choose natural beauty products.

If you are ready to get rid of those chemical-laden cosmetic products and enter the world of natural beauty, there are quite a few choices out there. You can often save money by making your own cosmetic products at home out of common kitchen goods. When you first begin a regimen of natural products, your body may go through a brief detoxifying period while it adjusts to not being drenched with toxins on a daily basis.

The face is often more sensitive than the skin on the rest of the body and must be treated accordingly. Look for a cleanser that does not dry the skin and is not too harsh. Castile soap or glycerin both work very well for cleaning the face without robbing it of precious moisture. Whatever type of cleanser you choose, be sure not to let your skin become dry and cracked, as this can lead to wrinkles.

Adding exfoliation to your daily skin care routine can help boost your skin's vibrancy and vitality.

Exfoliating removes the top layer of dead skin that accumulates over time. This dead material can choke off the oxygen and sunlight to the healthy skin below and gives your face a dull appearance. Exfoliating before cleansing will strip off this unnecessary layer and let your natural beauty shine through.

Always keep your skin protected from the damaging rays of the sun. Direct sunlight can burn out the pigmentation in certain spots of the skin, leading to unsightly age spots and white patches. There are many natural sunscreens available today, many of them consisting of simple ingredients like olive oil. Of course, staying out of the sun is your best bet, but a natural beauty product with sun protection can limit the damage if you must go out.

Natural hair coloring is also available as a healthier alternative to chemical-based dyes. Throughout history, natural products have been used to spice up appearance by changing hair color. Natural hair colorings give you the option of a more mellow, subtle color change or a more drastic change, depending on the material used as a dye. Using a tea rinse gives that nice, gentle look and something like henna can give you a brighter color that really pops.

It can be confusing at first, but making the change to natural beauty products is well worth the effort. It is easy to find information these days, with the accessibility of the Internet. Local health food stores or even pharmacies may have the latest natural cosmetic products as well. With so many options, there is no reason to continue using chemical-based commercial products instead of those that bring out your natural beauty.

Learn How to Make Natural Beauty Products at Home

Want to know how to make natural beauty products at home? There are a number of natural beauty recipes you can prepare with just a few items you may already have in your kitchen. Not only are these products easy to make, but they are also healthier than using commercial products full of chemicals.

By learning how to make natural beauty products of your own, you will be helping the environment, along with saving money. Most of the commercial cosmetic products on the market include some type of chemical or detergent. When this is washed off your skin or thrown in the trash, these chemicals and toxins can get into the water supply. Making your own natural beauty products out of common household items is a much greener solution.

Some common kitchen items that can be used to make natural beauty products are Epsom salt, bananas, honey, oatmeal, olive and vegetable oils, yogurt, mayonnaise. This is just a short list of household products that can be used for skin or hair care. There are quite a few other natural products that can do wonders for your appearance.

There are two common ingredients that you probably will not have on hand when you are learning how to make natural beauty products. These are beeswax and natural soap bars. Beeswax and other natural waxes can be found at health food stores, soap making shops, and some craft stores. For those allergic to bees, there are other vegetable- and flower-based waxes to choose from.

Olive oil is a very versatile home remedy that can be used for a number of natural beauty purposes. It will moisturize the dry skin of your elbows, cuticles, knees, and feet. Olive oil can be added to a warm bath for even more moisture and softness. For dry hair or scalp, simply massage the oil directly in with your hands.

You can even make your own natural exfoliating treatment from olive oil. Mix the oil with twice as much brown sugar to create a thick paste. Use this paste as a pre-shower skin treatment by rubbing gently into the skin. Rinse thoroughly in the shower to remove all paste and any dead skin cells that may have been scraped off.

If you have bananas on hand, you can also use those as a moisturizer for dry and cracked skin. Mash a ripe banana until it becomes a paste that is smooth enough to apply to your face or hands. Let the paste soak in for about ten minutes, then rinse off and pat dry. For added moisturizing, add in a teaspoon of olive oil before applying to dry, parched skin.

These are just a few of the beauty products you can make at home without spending much money. Other great home remedies include facial cleansers, herbal bath soaks, skin butter, and natural body scrubs.

Most of these recipes can be made with simple ingredients that you already have at home. Now that you know how easy it is, jump right in and learn how to make natural beauty products of your own.

Proven Skin Care Tips to Keep You Looking Young

If you're looking to prevent premature aging and look your absolute best, these skin care tips are for you. Of course, wrinkles are an inevitable part of getting older, but there are a few steps you can take to stay looking young as long as possible.

Keeping a healthy lifestyle is the best thing you can do for your skin. It starts with diet and nutrition as this is what fuels your body and provides nutrients to make essential oils and collagen for the skin. Fruits and vegetables are especially good for your body and skin because they contain fiber and antioxidants. Eat more healthy oils like olive oil and whole grains to provide nutrition without excess calories.

In addition to maintaining a proper food intake, drinking enough water is one of the most important skin care tips. Water will keep the skin moist and supply, while also clearing out toxins. Dry skin is extremely susceptible to wrinkles and fine lines, so you want to always stay hydrated. The standard recommendation is to drink six to eight glasses of water each day, whether or not you are trying to lose weight.

Regular exercise is also important to keep your skin healthy and vibrant. Exercise increases blood flow and helps clean out the pores by sweating out toxins.

Frequent physical activity will also improve your mood, enhance your cognitive skills, and reduce weight.

Reduce stress whenever possible as it can have an effect on your skin. Under stress, the body's metabolism is disrupted, which can lead to the signs of premature aging. Some good ways to relax and relieve stress include taking a bath, exercising, or meditation.

We all know how dangerous the sun's UV rays are, so always protect yourself when you go outside. The sun can dry out your skin's oils and natural moisture, making it more likely to crack or wrinkle. SPF 15 is standard protection, but fair-skinned people may need even more protection.

Other skin care tips include using jojoba oil or coenzyme Q10 to reduce wrinkles and protect your skin. Jojoba oil is a very versatile oil that can be used to reduce wrinkles, relax stretch marks, and provide moisture to dry, cracked skin. It is also very similar to some of the oils naturally produced by the skin, so it is tolerated well by the body.

Jojoba oil is very high in vitamin E, which is known to be an antioxidant that can help protect the skin from damage. Coenzyme Q10 is another popular anti-wrinkle ingredient. It is mostly used for its antioxidant properties, which protect the skin cells from free radicals. Free radicals are continually generated by the body's metabolic processes and will break down the structure of the cell. Since they are always being created by the body, a daily antioxidant is necessary to keep free radicals under control.

Now you know several easy ways to protect yourself from the signs of premature aging.

Look for anti-wrinkle products containing the ingredients listed above to make sure you are getting a quality product. Stay consistent in following our skin care tips and you will find yourself looking younger each day.

Sakura®
Nutraceuticals

ADVANCED PRODUCTS BACKED BY: NATURE+SCIENCE

www.SakuraNutraceuticals.com

Simple Safe Acne Anti-Aging Skin Care

Are you facing the problem of your skin aging before it's time? Relax! Thanks to the advances in acne anti-aging skin care treatments there is a skin care product or actual medical treatment to help you. However, you and I need to know a few things before we can choose the right skin care treatment.

As a matter of course, before you or I even think about what product or type of treatment we are going to employ, we should always consult a qualified professional first. Obviously, the well trained and licensed physician can advise us as to what our actual skin problems are.

Many times, we may find out that we have an underlying health condition, such as a thyroid problem or other condition, causing our skin to age faster than normal. Obviously, treating the medical problem would be the very first step in our battle; to stop the premature aging of our skin. In addition to ruling out a medical condition, there are a few other things our doctor will be able to fill us in on.

One of the first things we need to know is that, as in many other things, female and male skin is different.

Big surprise! Right? As an example a man's face, when treating over exposure to the sun, wind and other environmental hazards, needs a skin care moisturizer which contains vitamin B5. Many of today's dermatologists also recommend creams with a combination of witch hazel and B5.

However, because the fairer sex, have other problems with their skin, than the old rugged male, women only need B5 in their acne anti-aging skin care battle. But it really helps both men and women, to kick their skin care battle up a notch, to include lotions and moisturizer creams with vitamins such as coenzyme Q10. In addition there are many other ingredients found in today's moisturizer creams and lotions.

A great many of the over the counter lotions and moisturizer creams contain an ingredient known as petrolatum. Emphasis on the petro! Because it is so common many of us have used it for years and guess what?

Yep! You guessed it. It may cause our skin to age that much faster. Studies which have been conducted, over the years, by well qualified skin specialist; bear this theory out. One of the easiest and simplest things to do in our acne anti-aging skin care treatment; is to avoid the products which contain petrolatum. But we need to remember there are other chemical and preservatives which should be avoided.

We should take the time to read every label on every bottle and tube of skin treatment products. However you and I know, we normally can't spell many of the ingredients listed, much less pronounce them or know what they mean.

Here's a little tip, a science teacher friend of mine gave me. If the word is about 2 inches long, chances are it is a chemical compound which is not natural to our body. Avoid it!

It's easy for us to understand there is more to simple, safe acne anti-aging skin care than just using any old cream or moisturizer. It will pay for us to gain as much knowledge as we can; to keep us from looking old before our time.

The Best Natural Beauty Recipes

There are a number of natural beauty recipes you can make at home. You do not have to pay for commercial cosmetic products to look your best. In fact, many times the natural solution is healthier and more effective than the chemical-laden make-ups you will find at the store.

Here is a great papaya enzyme facial mask that is one of the more popular natural beauty recipes. You will need the following ingredients: 1/2 cup mashed papaya, 1 whipped egg white, and 1 teaspoon of honey. For additional cooling or if you have sensitive skin, add a tablespoon of plain yogurt to your mixture.

Mix all of your ingredients together in a large bowl. Wash your skin before applying the facial mask mixture. Leave the mask on your face for approximately five to eight minutes, giving the papaya enzymes time to exfoliate your skin. Rinse off with warm water first, then with cooler water, patting dry when done.

For hair, this herbal vinegar rinse will restore your hair's natural pH balance, clean off built up dirt and hair products, and reduce oily hair. Place 2 sprigs of rosemary and 2 sprigs of lavender in 2 cups of water in a clear glass jar. Let the jar sit out in the sun to steep for between two and four hours, then remove the herbs. Add one or two tablespoons of either apple cider vinegar or white vinegar to your water solution, then use the same way you would use shampoo.

Herbal bath salts are another of the top natural beauty recipes you can make at home. All you need is a cup of sea salt and a handful of whatever herbs you have on hand, such as lavender, rosemary, spearmint, or peppermint. Grind the herbs with a coffee grinder until they become a fine powder. Mix with the sea salt and dump into your next bath for a relaxing change of pace.

A similar natural beauty recipe is this refreshing flower-based foot soak. For this one, you again need sea salt, along with some fresh sliced citrus of your choice (limes, lemons, oranges, etc.) and a handful of flower petals picked fresh from your garden. Fill a small basin with lukewarm water and add the salt, flower petals, and fruit slices. Soak your feet in the mixture for ten minutes, then rinse and pat to dry.

This strawberry manicure mask is a great way to pamper your hands naturally. Mash 3-5 ripe strawberries, drain off the juice, and combine with one tablespoon of sugar and a little bit of the light oil of your choice. Apply the resulting mixture to your hands by using a circular motion. This will condition and exfoliate the skin, leaving it soft and smooth.

During watermelon season, this pedicure polish is good for your feet and gives your home a nice aroma of summer. Combine 1/2 cup of mashed and strained watermelon with one tablespoon finely crushed almonds and 1/4 cup of plain yogurt. Apply the mixture by working it in with your hands in a circular motion. Use a tissue to remove, then rinse and pat dry to enjoy this one of our natural beauty recipes.

What You Need to Know About Organic Skin Care

Because today's consumers are more conscious of their health and the environment, there are more organic skin care products available than ever before. Other people may have developed allergies to all of the toxins and chemicals used in commercial skin care products and are looking for a healthier alternative. Some commonly used ingredients in commercial products include fragrances, dyes, and various types of acids.

By contrast, organic skin care products contain natural ingredients such as vitamins A, C, or E, essential oils, antioxidants, or proteins. These are necessary to replace the skin cells lost as we age. As the body gets older, it produces less collagen and elastin, which leads to dry, wrinkled skin. Re-hydrating the cells from the outside is the only way to repair this age-related damage.

You can now find organic skin care products in almost any pharmacy, drug store, or health food and nutrition store. If you do not have access to any of these places, there are many retailers online to choose your natural cosmetics from.

Some spas and salons have also added organic products to their inventory, so you may want to look there as well. Most of these products are free of fragrances and dyes and will not cause or aggravate existing allergies.

There are organic products available both men and women. Men can find organic shaving lotion and after-shave, while women usually have more options of cleansers, creams, toners, and gels.

Unfortunately, organic products generally cost more than the synthetic version of the same item. It is worth the extra cost to protect your skin and your health from toxic chemicals and preservatives.

An alarming number of mainstream skin care products may contain the wetting agents diethanolamine and triethanolamine, sometimes listed on ingredient labels as DEA and TEA, respectively. These substances by themselves are not considered to be a cancer risk.

If the product contains nitrites as contaminants, this may cause a chemical reaction that creates cancer-causing nitrosamines.

Most commercial cosmetic products include some type of bactericides or preservatives. These are necessary to protect the cosmetics from contamination, but may also be dangerous or even carcinogenic.

For instance, trace amounts of formaldehyde are found in some products. Formaldehyde is a known carcinogen and is neurotoxic in higher doses.

How can you be sure that your skin care products are really organic? Unfortunately, there is still plenty of room for vagueness in labeling of cosmetic products. Generally, a cosmetic product must follow the same USDA rules as would a food product.

The product must contain no less than 95% organic and natural ingredients in order to qualify for the label.

After the 95% threshold is met, there is a serious lack of additional guidance and regulations. There are no restrictions on the words cosmetic manufacturers can use on their labels, so you many see plenty of products called "organic" or "botanical" even though they may still contain a small amount of synthetic chemicals.

Read the ingredient labels carefully to be sure that your organic skin care products are really made of only organic materials.

Why You Should Try All Natural Skin Care Products

Wondering about all natural skin care products? There are a lot of choices on the market today and it can be confusing when you are trying to decide which products are best for you. Here are a few things to consider before shopping for a new skin care program.

Environmental pollution and sun exposure can increase production of free radicals in the body. The body already produces these skin-damaging free radicals on a continual basis during the process of metabolism. Free radicals can cause mutations in the skin cells that may lead to cancer or, at the very least, premature wrinkles. All good skin care programs should include some form of sun protection.

Most all natural skin care products do contain sunscreen, so check the label for the level of SPF protection. Be careful if you are using sunblock every time you are in the sun because this may cause a vitamin D deficiency. To be safe, supplement your nutritional intake with a daily multivitamin.

Lack of vitamin D has been connected to osteoporosis, so older women should be extra careful to replace their vitamin intake.

There has been a recent trend toward more nutrition-related skin care products. Poor diet and bad physical health does affect the skin cells, as well as the rest of the body. Vitamin C is especially good for skin health and may even prevent some damage caused by sun exposure.

Antioxidant vitamins remove free radicals, which can damage skin cells and lead to premature aging. Our body is always producing free radicals as a byproduct of metabolism, so a daily antioxidant vitamin supplement can be very helpful.

Honey is an excellent material for all natural skin care products because it can lock in moisture that is already present in the skin. Many spas used paraffin wax in the past for this purpose, but now it is recognized that honey is a much more useful natural alternative.

Vegetable oil and natural waxes will also have this effect if you would rather not use honey or do not have any available.

Honey is not a very effective natural moisturizer because it does not contain any water. However, it does not dry out the skin the way alcohol and other common cosmetic ingredients might. Honey can also inhibit bacterial growth and other acne-causing organisms.

There are specialized honeys available for use as all-natural skin care products, which are significantly different than the honey you would find at the store.

Another kitchen item that can be found in the best all natural skin care products is olive oil. Olive oil has a variety of uses in natural cosmetics, including moisturizing the skin or hair. It can be used on the dry, parched skin found on the heels, elbows, or knees.

Throw a little bit of olive oil into your next bath for added softness and luxury. Olive oil can even moisturize the hair and scalp if rubbed directly on the head.

Olive oil also makes a nice natural exfoliant for the skin. Simply mixing some oil with a quantity of brown sugar will create a thick exfoliant paste. The paste can then be used before a shower or bath as an exfoliating treatment.

Olive oil is just one example of the great all-natural skin care products that can be used to moisturize and protect your skin.

Cheat Sheet for Being Beautiful

All the Low Down on The Newest Products for Physical Beauty

Body Products Basics

It's easy to jam your cosmetic bag with things you believe you have to have, however one thing we seem to forget is the basics. If you don't attend to your skin no amount of expensive make-up will help make you look unflawed. Begin from the basic skincare products like exfoliates and cleansers. An exceptional moisturizer is a must. In addition to that, if you plan to put make-up on, don't blank out taking it off. A gentle make-up remover, particularly an eye make-up remover is suggested.

The Basics

Likewise, purchase little product sizes or trial sizes when you are able to. This will let you try the product on and see if it matches with your skin, and you are able to easily substitute it without dropping a lot of cash. I particularly abide by this rule when it comes to cleansers, moisturizers and make-up removers. Anything that annoys my skin is directly removed as it's too harsh and isn't well-matched with my sensitive skin.

Facial Cleanser Tip

Simply like the rest of your body, your face has to have a good wash also. I keep my face cleaner in the shower, that way I may wash my face as I shower. This, also as the cleansing right after your shower technique, is suggested because your pores will be more open and your face will get a deeper cleaning.

Find products that are natural and plant derived. These products are gentle and may be utilized for oily to normal skin. Their key ingredients are Camomile, Lavender, Rosemary, Vitamin E.

Your skin will be smooth and the cleanser is amazing for sensitive skin.

This cleanser needs to be gentle enough to be utilized on an everyday basis. Make sure it bears no potentially skin-irritating detergents. It is a self-foaming cleaner, even though it doesn't utilize the standard foam components. These products remove every speck of dirt, particularly eye makeup. You won't walk out of the shower looking like a raccoon after washing off your face with these cleansers. Another thing to keep in the shower is a battery-operated cleanser that comes with its own cleansing pads or you are able to utilize it with your preferred cleanser. The first time you use it, it will feel like two layers of dead skin come off your my face.

Find a great moisturizer or skin cream. Find one that is lightweight and may be worn without any make-up over it. This will help to reduce signs of fine lines. After a time of using such products you ought to notice glowing and radiant skin.

Silky smooth primer coat is a must prior to your foundation. This product will cover up any skin imperfections, fill out fine lines and cut down the appearance of pores. It will make your foundation go on swimmingly and perfect, resulting in durable make-up. I've discovered this product to make my skin appear unflawed in pictures also.

I hope these general beauty products help get you started to beautiful, beaming skin. Remember that no amount of expensive make-up will look great unless you have fresh and clear skin underneath.

Be Educated on Toxins and Detoxing

What are toxins, and how do they develop in my body? What are the facts?

Detox! If you're like me, you listen to statement like these from a lot of wellness-minded folks:

"I have to free my body of toxins, time to detox."

"I'm beginning a detox diet this week."

"Time for my yearly detox juice fast!"

I'm fit, how come I have to 'Detox'? A lot of us work hard to consume the correct foods, practice health strategies and observe our tension levels. However even the fittest of people tend to sweep up 'detox practices'. Are body toxins real? Doesn't our body attend to toxins on our own? What are toxins that develop in my body?

Detox: "Toxins" while almost sounding like an urban myth, are indeed real.

A toxin is a chemical or poison that's understood to have adverse effects on the body. Toxins might come from food or water, from chemicals utilized to grow or fix food, and even from the air that we breathe. Our bodies treat those toxins through body organs like the liver and kidneys and excrete them in the form of sweat, urine, and fecal matter.

You might break toxins down into 4 classes: toxins from the air, water, food and chemicals in our surroundings. Here is an illustration of each:

Air: Pollution denotes the toxic gases and chemicals, like methane and carbon monoxide gas that are released into the air only to be blended into the air we breathe in and breathe out. Pollution toxins might come from vehicle and factory emissions as well as additional sources. A notable air pollutant is likewise cigarettes. Breathed in tobacco products contain a measure of extremely toxic ingredients that could negatively affect your body.

Water: A list of toxins has been found in water. Everything from chlorine, bleach, ammonium hydroxide and even OTC and prescription drugs have been reported to be detected in excess in drinking water. Pollutants and chemicals in water have been stated to cause everything from depressive disorder to sickness and even cancer.

Water systems across the world greatly vary in composition. Spring, mineral and artisan bottled waters have gotten to be all the rage in the past decade, though some critics consider that tap water isn't as bad as the media depicts.

Food: toxic foods don't refer to pesticides. Toxic foods might refer to artificial additives, extremely processed or genetically altered foods and even chemical components in food recipes like food dyes and chemical flavorings.

Some physicians think that modern day American diets might really be considered 'toxic' because of the high consumption of processed, dead 'empty-calorie' food items like white flour and sugar.

Chemicals: Chemicals that are toxic might include little amounts of really toxic things, like pesticide residue dusted onto our newly - picked, non-washed, non-organic produce. Elevated pesticide produce items include non-organic peaches, strawberries, apples, nectarines, sweet peppers, celery, cherries, lettuce, imported grapes and pears. Nonprescription, prescription and even recreational drugs are all denoted as chemical toxins that might build up in your body over time.

Why should I 'detox' my body?

The general idea behind a 'detox diet or regimen' is that the contemporary world places so much stress on our bodies as we are exposed to a multitude of toxins on a day-to-day basis, and the natural detoxification mechanisms in place in our bodies can't keep up the detox demands. Consequently, 'active detox' is a good idea. "Detoxing" refers to taking additional measures to guarantee that your body detoxes properly-to deter any damaging effects of toxin-build-up in your body.

Does my body detox by nature? Our bodies are bright. They've built in mechanisms to detox 'toxins'. Detox organs include: liver, kidneys, skin and lungs. Our bodies' digestive, lymphatic and cardiovascular system all plays a chief role in the procedure of detox.

What is assisted detox?

Detox diets, fasting and cleanse diets might refer to a few things: super- high intake of 'colon-cleansing' fiber, intended to literally brush and sweep out the developed toxins in your colon. A different detox method is 'fasting'. A fasting is an ultra-low-calorie diet (occasionally in all-liquid form) meant to take the strain off your digestive system for a few hours, days or weeks so to pump up the natural detoxing powers of your body.

Skin Detox. A different form of detox help might come through the skin: sweat rooms and 'hot yoga' provide high-sweat surroundings meant to accelerate detox through the biggest organ in your body- skin. Epsom salts and 'skin brushing' are health practices that have likewise been shown to accelerate the detox of skin-bound toxins.

There are indeed a lot of false-claim products and dangerous/hazardous practices out there to pick from. And as a matter of fact, many 'fasts' and 'detox diets' might be harmful to particular people. "Serious Fasting" is something that ought to be attempted only under the watch of a physician or dietitian. A softer organic juice-raw food 'fast or diet' might be a beneficial way for healthy folks to help the detox process. However again, any 'fast' isn't to be taken lightly.

How to detox by nature and healthfully?

One innate, extremely effective and safe form of 'detox enhancement' is workouts! Exercise quickens your circulatory and respiratory systems and raises natural sweating-all natural detox techniques utilized by the body (lungs, skin and blood/gastrointestinal system).

A different really crucial part of natural detox is your hydration level! Your body will detox itself much easier if you're totally hydrated. Water, fresh fruit juices, herb tea, kombucha and coconut water are fabulous drinks to remain hydrated.

And finally, massage is a natural way to accelerate detox. By kneading your body muscles and skin, you're loosening the toxins that are stored or 'building' in your cells.

Professional athletes frequently partake in everyday massages to relax their muscles and one theory is to loosen the lactic acid brought on by exercise- possibly the reason for sore muscles. Overall, massages are one technique that might help you naturally detox. And incentive, a massage feels amazing!

Using Bath Products

Suitable bathing is the much for a beautiful body otherwise beauty is incomplete. Bathing is the sole thing which one does to prettify the whole body. It's simply not a routine of the day but has gotten to be a luxury also.

Even in ancient times baths, tubs and spas were there with all the world's most luxurious items involved for the bath. Nowadays individuals invest an equal amount and time in getting a bath done as they do for the additional parts of the home.

There are particular basics for the perfect bath and bathroom, which haven't changed even though the time has shifted. They're just the same as ancient times where hygiene was regarded as the chief priority of a bath and the bathroom.

The Bath

The bath ought to be neat and clean. Even though it's not roomy, you may make it that way by keeping everything as soaps, shampoos, oils, lotions and towel's in place. Even if you've a huge bathroom with all the luxuries like bathtub, sauna but you keep is messy then it cuts down on the advantages. You yourself won't enjoy using it.

Keep the towels clean and dry and do not share your towel with other people. It's not hygienic and can pass on the infections. If you do not air dry the towels, they may get a musty smell and leave a bad odor in the bathroom.

Keep a foot mat in the bath to soak the water and wipe off the feet.

Keep your bathing accouterments like loofahs, scrubber and sponge clean. Wash them in running hot water, squeeze them, and do not leave water and soap inside them. Do not share them with other people to prevent skin infections.

Clean the bath with antiseptic and put scented flowers and additional items in the room to make it smell fresh and clean.

Replace your brushes, loofah and sponge every alternate month for best hygiene.

These are simple ways for a beauty bath-if you do not have luxuries like bathing tub or spa in your bathroom.

Massage your body with vitamin E or olive oil. Take your shower. Shampoo and condition your hair if you do it daily. Wash yourself clean. Dry off with dry towel. Now apply body lotion all over your body. Use deodorant or roll on stick to smell good. You ought to always pick out your soap depending upon your skin type and weather. Moisturizing soaps are more beneficial in winter, whereas antiseptics are great in summers to prevent heat boils and sweat.

You may apply readymade or homemade body scrubs to increase the body's blood circulation get rid of the dead skin cells and give your bath a memorable experience. If you do not have time to apply a body pack or scrub every day, you may do it once a week. Readymade scrubs are available at any cosmetic shop. Here are few homemade body scrubs, which you may make simply at home and apply on your face and body.

The easiest and oldest homemade body scrub is made by wheat flour and curd. Take some wheat flour in a bowl, add a pinch of turmeric to it, and make a paste of it by putting in curd. Apply it on the body and scrub it off once it's half dry. It will polish off dead skin make it glowing and blemish free.

Soak rice overnight in milk. Grind it in a mixture and make a paste, scrub it all over the body. This scrub removes the black and white heads from your body and makes it polished.

You may add rose petals to your bath water to make pleasant aromatics.

You may purchase scented aroma oils to relax and soothe your mind and body. They're added in the bath water.

If you get heat boils on your body in summers, add a mug of boiled neem leave's water in your bath water every day to get rid of them.

Utilize a paste of sandalwood powder all over your body in summer to prevent heat infections on the skin, to smell great and control oil on the skin.

Take normal wheat flour. Add raw milk to it. Apply this paste all over your body and rub it off in the opposite direction. This removes small excessive hair from your body and makes the skin polished.
You may boil orange and lemon peels in water. Let it cool and then mix it in your bath water. You'll feel fresh throughout the day.

Sunless Tanning

Don't wish to expose your skin to the sun's damaging rays, but don't wish to miss out on that sun-kissed glow? Think about affecting a compromise with sunless tanning products. Begin by comprehending how sunless tanning products work — and the significance of utilizing them right and carefully.

Tanning

Sunless tanning products, likewise known as self-tanners, may give your skin a suntanned look without exposing it to adverse ultraviolet (UV) rays. Sunless bronzing products are generally sold as creams, gels, lotions and sprays you put on your skin. Pro spray-on tanning likewise is available at a lot of salons, spas and tanning businesses.

The active ingredient in many sunless tanning products is dihydroxyacetone (DHA). When put on to the skin, DHA responds with dead cells in the outermost layer of skin to temporarily darken the skin's appearance. The color doesn't wash off; however it gradually disappears as the dead skin cells shed off — commonly within a few days.

Many sunless tanning products don't contain sun blocker. If you spend time outside, sun blocker remains crucial.

What about sunless tanning pills?

Sunless tanning pills, which commonly contain the coloration additive canthaxanthin, are dangerous. If taken in big amounts, canthaxanthin may turn your skin orange and induce hives. Sunless tanning pills may likewise induce liver damage and lead to the formation of crystals in the retina of the eye (canthaxanthin retinopathy).

What may you expect from sunless tanning products?

Sunless tanning products commonly go on clear. It commonly takes approximately an hour to see results. Full color commonly comes along within 8 to 24 hours. Individuals who have medium skin color without freckles frequently get the most beneficial results.

Is sunless tanning dependable?

Topical sunless tanning products are commonly considered safe options to sunbathing, as long as they're utilized as directed.

Bear in mind that spray-on tanning or mist-on tanning from a beauty parlor or spa is commonly applied to all parts of your body, including your face, to guarantee an even color.

This produces a potential for the product to get in and around your eyes, near your nostrils or onto your lips. The hazards, if any, of breathing in or ingesting DHA are obscure — so close your eyes and hold your breath while the tanner is put on.

You might likewise need to request or bring along protective devices, like goggles or nose plugs.

What's the most beneficial way to advance an even-looking tan with sunless tanning products?

Sunless tanning products may supply an even, natural-looking tan if they're put on right and carefully. For most beneficial results, abide by the package directions carefully. At large:

Exfoliate first. Prior to utilizing a sunless tanning product, wash your skin with a wash cloth or sponge to take away excess dead skin cells. If you commonly shave your legs, do so prior to applying the sunless tanning product for an even application.

Utilize a light touch. Put on the sunless tanning product evenly and thinly. Utilize sparingly on dry or thickened skin, like over your ankles, knees and elbows. If necessary, ask somebody to help you put on sunless tanner to hard-to-reach spots.

Save the tops of your hands for last. After you apply the product to your face and body, rinse your hands with soap and water to prevent coloring your palms. Make sure to remove any product from below your fingernails. Then utilize a cotton ball to apply the sunless tanner to the top of each hand.

Take time to dry. Wait to dress till the sunless tanner dries totally.

Remember, many sunless tanning products don't carry sun blocker. If you spend time outside, protect your skin with generous amounts of sun block.

Body Makeup

With more skin showing this season, a few of us might be a bit concerned with our exposed body parts not appearing so perfect. As we mature, veins, sunspots, freckles and easy bruising might be an issue. Do not put away your tanks or minis just yet. There are a couple of fast and simple ways to conceal so you are able to reveal.

Make-up for The Body

First of all, consider utilizing a subtle self-tanner. This alone might be all you have you have to cover up minor imperfections on the skin so you are able to show off your body with confidence. Try Jerkens Natural Glow for a really light way to fake the suntan. If you're seeking more of a bronze goddess gleam, attempt going to a spray tanning beauty salon for a pro job.

You are able to likewise apply a makeup bronzer to your skin to produce the same effect. It's great if you don't need something permanent — you are able to simply wash it off at the finish of the night. Try out one like Laura Mercier Body Bronzing Makeup, which bears light reflecting particles that will bounce light off imperfections and supply you a nice color at the same time.

If little veins or sun spots on your chest are a true issue, or if you merely need more coverage, attempt using a spray foundation. Sally Hansen Natural Beauty quickly and softly covers up unsightly defects and produces a smooth look. Merely spray directly onto the skin then utilize a non-latex sponge to buff it in. It goes on transparent, dries easy, is water-resistant and won't rub off on apparel.

For varicose veins, bruises or birthmarks on the legs you ought to apply a little concealer. Merely dab concealer over the area with a small-tipped concealer brush and utilize a light dusting of powder to set. I enjoy Amazing Cosmetics Concealer as it has an exceptional consistency and its waterproof so it will last all day — even at the beach.

So don’t worry about defects and flaunt that chassis!

The Latest in Support Garments

A wardrobe is part of each woman's life. There's more to a woman's wardrobe than simply skirts, dresses, pants and blouses. There are underclothes. There might have been a day when one undergarment fit each occasion but that day is long gone.

Underwear

Today's well put together woman has an underclothes wardrobe simply as voluminous as her over clothes wardrobe. It has to begin with a couple of common pieces and from that a wardrobe can be built. The bra is a basic of any woman's underclothes wardrobe. White and black are the general colors for woman's bras however flesh colored is likewise a basic that's necessary to wear under blouses and shirts that are sheer. The sort of bra will be influenced by the breast size of the woman.

At least one bra needs to be of a material that will supply the coverage essential to wear under a T-shirt regardless what the temperature. A bra with additional support works well for big breasted women and a demi-cup or push up bra is the perfect basic for a littler chested woman.

The basic bra wardrobe ought to begin with at least 4 bras.

- A T-shirt bra
- A dress bra
- A sport bra
- An adjustable strap bra

Panties are a different staple of a basic underclothes wardrobe. First make sure your panties fit right. Ill-fitting panties will show through apparel and the look isn't attractive. It doesn't matter as you like thongs, bikinis, hipsters or wide-cut panties, if you see the panty line, it's incorrect.

White and black are the common panty colors. Flesh color is likewise a great choice since it is not visible through even the filmiest material. The general panty wardrobe ought to include:

- A pair of white and or black
- A pair of flesh color
- A pair of support panties
- A pair of no line panties

With the new filmy and clinging fabrics, Spanx are a woman's most beneficial friend. These are underclothes however they go over your traditional underclothes to keep everything together and to prevent the jiggle that any additional inches may supply. It isn't simply for bigger woman; each woman has some curves that may take away from that perfect sleek and brushed up look and Spanx provides a tiny bit of additional support.

An underbodice is a light weight undergarment that's worn underneath a sheer blouse or shirt.

The general wardrobe will have at least one and the color will be fixed by the blouse it's to be worn with.

A slip is the perfect undergarment to wear with a shirt or a dress particularly whenever the skirt or dress is made of a filmy or clinging material. The general colors are white, black and flesh colored. The general slip wardrobe consists of:

- A total slip
- A one-half slip

Don't ever get caught up with the improper underclothes. Simply follow these simple rules and you'll be prepared for each occasion. Firstly you have to think that your underclothes ought to always compliment.

Getting your right measurements is critical when it comes to underclothes it’s like recognizing your shoe size you wouldn't purchase a pair of shoes that was a size to big or too little and you for sure shouldn't do the same with your underclothes.

You are able to go to most any department store and ask them about acquiring your measurements and most of the time it's free of charge. When you don't feel easy doing that utilize your our measuring tape at home around your breasts, your tummy holding the tape at your navel, and your hips going around the broadest part of your butt.

Comfort is the most crucial factor in selecting great underclothes you are able to find something comfy in each style when you’re willing to look hard enough, so know which fabrics you like best and, on many occasions, limit yourself to them.

When you're curious how a g-string or a thong will work for you purchase yourself a cheap pair and wear them around your house one day while you're doing housekeeping. That's a great true test to see when they'll work for you.

Pairing your bra with your panties may be a nice way to ramp up your self-assurance in an outfit. It is after all about authority here ladies and when we know we have sexy matching underclothes set on underneath it demonstrates in our step.

It's crucial that you own both bras and panties in a mass of colors. Your clothes are not all one color why should your underclothes be. Black underclothes aren't taboo it's bold and confident, so don't be frightened to purchase something in red, pink, purple, and any colors you're into. For the plus size ladies out there Lane Bryant makes their bigger underclothes in colored plus sizes unlike other stores that solely carry white, black, and tan in their plus lines.

When you're into lace get yourself something lacy in a racy color likewise with silk, cotton, etc. You know what's underneath and there's nothing sexier to a man than undressing his love and discovering another present waiting below.

I urge every woman to do their greater investing in their bras as a great bra may be very versatile among your outfits and there's nothing sorrier than a cheap bra that's wires start to break out after a couple of washings.
I'd say twenty-five bucks or more is what you ought to be expecting to spend.

Many department stores have separate lingerie departments where you'll discover all the designers and selections. Bear in mind for that budget shopper that the clearance section in lingerie department isn't like the one in other departments, the seasons change quickly with underclothes and they put everything on their clearance rack not simply the size extra small.

And last but surely not least...know your designers! Each designer varies in the size section so occasionally your typical medium may fit like a small or a large so try them on and make your modifications accordingly.

When you abide by these easy rules you'll be a pro in the underclothes department in no time.

How Looking Great Makes You Feel Great

I know, I understand, beauty is superficial. However still, looking great makes me feel great. I get a total feeling of self-assurance when I look great. Dressing up appears to put me in a great mood contrary to those scrubbed out, gloomy, pessimistic days.

In my judgment, if what's on the outside looks even as great as what's on the inside, it will be almost effortless for your glowing personality to come out and for the world to see just how amazing you truly are.

Advantages

Here are some reasons why looking great makes me feel great:

1. I get a self-boost. Everybody needs one once in a while. It's that feeling of, "Damn I look great!" that gives me reassurance that yes I'm that exceptional (and so are you!).

2. Individuals tell me I look great. This makes me satisfied because regardless how many times I tell myself not to care what other people think, it does help to hear that they like what I've done with myself. You tell me what makes you feel better--positive regard or bad glares?

3. I feel like I may achieve anything. I look exceptional so why not do exceptional things? Looking great gives me that additional spark to get things going and make a difference in the world.

4. Individuals talk to me. I'm not trying to say that other individuals have no friends, however from natural observation, it's the ill groomed kids who had no one to play with during recess, who were commonly sitting alone in the cafeteria, and who were so shy they may barely get through the day.

5. Here's the resolution: take pride in your outer look and the power to socialize will become much easier. When you look pretty and accessible, individuals will draw close to you.

6. it's amusing. I like getting ready and looking great--putting on pretty outfits, styling my hair, and putting on makeup. This makes me satisfied, and being satisfied is an exceptional way for me to feel great.

Wrapping Up

So, what is true beauty? It sure isn't a mystical ingredient in ultra-long-lasting lip gloss, and you certainly won't discover it hidden in the cosmetics aisle at the pharmacy.

It's the knowledge that you love yourself, and that you're true to your own heart. It's having eyes that glitter with compassion and see the best in individuals. It's bearing lips that speak strongly when you've been bossed around and gently when somebody else has been.

The most beautiful trait you are able to have is self-assurance! Work out what you like about yourself and let it glow. That's what true beauty is all about.

Sakura®
Nutraceuticals
ADVANCED PRODUCTS BACKED BY: NATURE+SCIENCE

Made in the USA
Monee, IL
04 November 2026

67387540R00066